PATIENT RELATED MULTIPLE CHOICE QUESTIONS
THE PATIENT WITH A GASTROINTESTINAL DISORDER

PATIENT RELATED MULTIPLE CHOICE QUESTIONS
QUESTIONS
THE PATIENT WITH A
GASTROINTESTINAL DISORDER

Anne Betts, SRN, RNT
Senior Tutor

Marjorie Read, BA, SRN, RNT, DipN
Assistant Director of Nurse Education

Maureen Theobald, SRN, RCNT, RNT, DipEd
Assistant Director of Nurse Education

The Princess Alexandra School of Nursing
The London Hospital
London

Cynthia Gilling, SRN, SCM, RNT
Director of Nurse Education
Royal Free Hospital
London

Harper & Row, Publishers
London

Cambridge		San Francisco
Hagerstown		Mexico City
Philadelphia		Sao Paulo
New York		Sydney

First published 1984

Harper & Row Ltd
28 Tavistock Street
London WC2E 7PN

British Library Cataloguing in Publication Data

Betts, Anne
　　Patient with a gastrointestinal disorder.—(Patient related
　　multiple choice questions)
　　1. Gastrointestinal system—Diseases—Problems, exercises,
　　etc.
　　I. Title　　II. Series
　　616.3′3′0024613　　RC801

　　ISBN 0-06-318254-8

Typeset by Gedset Limited, Cheltenham
Printed and bound by A. Wheaton & Co.

For Robert J. Read
and his 'technological' help, without which
the validation process would be even more painful

CONTENTS

Foreword   vi

Preface   vii

How to use this book   1

Patient-related multiple choice questions   4

Answers   73

FOREWORD

Anne Betts, Cynthia Gilling, Maureen Theobald and Marjorie Read are four senior teachers of nursing, working in the same school. As a result of much burning of the midnight oil and close collaboration, they have produced this fourth book in a series called *Patient-Related Multiple Choice Questions*. As teachers they are fully committed to the concept that learning is ongoing, largely self-directed, and that the continuing assessment of knowledge and understanding is an integral part of the learning process. This book, and the others in the series, will aid the nurse learner in a practical way to assess her own progress.

This series comes at a most appropriate time. The English National Board is currently reviewing the methods used to examine nurse learners to determine entry into the profession. Since 1983 there has been a change in the format of the multi-choice objective questions used in the State Written Examination and Assessment.

The patient-related stories used in this book will, hopefully, not only help nurse teachers produce their own valid questions, but also stimulate ideas and discussion between all nurses involved in the teaching of patient care. Methods of teaching, learning and assessing are vital components of the nursing curriculum, which should not be static. The development or modification of one part should therefore lead to the consideration of the validity of the others.

The value of this book will be in its practical use as an assessment tool, and in promoting a fresh look at current practices in nursing education.

The success of the series is evident in the total number of books which have been sold, and in the number of positive comments received by the authors from nurse learners and nurse teachers alike.

The problem-solving approach to individual patient care which is currently being developed in many schools of nursing requires methods of examining knowledge which promote debate and discussion. Multiple choice questions related to patient care is one of these methods, and the series of books provides a useful tool for nurse learners and their teachers.

Edith R. Parker, MSc, BA (Hons), SRN, RMN, SCM, RNT
1984

PREFACE

Multiple choice questions have become an established part of the State Examination system since 30 unrelated items were replaced by story-related questions in the final examinations in January 1983. The value of linking several questions together by relating them to a short story concerning a particular patient is also proven as a teaching tool. Questions provoke answers but multiple choice questions stimulate discussion to arrive at the answer, thus enhancing the problem-solving approach to patient-centred nursing. This aspect makes such an approach dual purpose in that it promotes learning as well as testing understanding.

Nurses in training are forever 'hungry' for more help, more practice and more stories. The problem is the relentlessness with which new stories need to be produced. Stories take a few minutes to answer but from our experience some hours to compose, shred, test and edit to make them valid and reliable.

The situation is improving as more and more tutors gain experience in producing more and more items and every contribution helps.

This series, of which this is the fourth book, is designed to be used by all nurses in training and is aimed at covering the applied principles of nursing care in a variety of settings with a variety of patients. Each book focuses on patients with conditions that may be similar but, because the patient's circumstances are different, a different nursing approach will be needed. We hope that it continues to meet the needs of learners.

The authors thank all those students at the St Bartholomew's School of Nursing and the Princess Alexandra School of Nursing, London, who have tested our items and offered their constructive criticism.

Anne Betts
Cynthia Gilling
Marjorie Read
Maureen Theobald

How to use this book

Each question starts with a brief 'story' about the patient, followed by a series of related multiple choice questions.

It will be necessary to refer back to the story when selecting your answer, bearing in mind the individuality of the patient and the need to assess the effect that this may have on the care planned.

It is our belief that there is only one right answer to each question, and we have given our reasons for selecting this as the most appropriate answer in a section at the end of the book.

EXAMPLE

Mrs Funmi Aghomi,   aged 34 years, is married with two children. She has not been feeling well recently but put it down to her recent pregnancy and her seeming increasing obesity. Nausea and vomiting and sore ribs made her visit her general practitioner where a diagnosis of infective hepatitis was made.

1 Which one of the following is *not* applicable to the aetiology of infective hepatitis?
   (a) it is a notifiable disease,
   (b) it is common where conditions of hygiene are poor,
   (c) hepatitis B surface antigen is associated with infective hepatitis,
   (d) the disease is transmitted principally by the faeco-oral route.

2 Which one of the following should Mrs Aghomi be advised to carry out by her general practitioner?
   (a) go home and go to bed,
   (b) isolate the family indoors for 5 days,
   (c) get ready some things for admission to hospital,
   (d) get plenty of rest and do less housework for the next 2 weeks.

3 Which of the following is the best reply to give Mrs Aghomi when she asks 'How long will I be jaundiced?'
   (a) it takes a long time to fade,
   (b) its difficult to say, but usually about 2 weeks or so,
   (c) jaundice develops rapidly and disappears as quickly as it comes,
   (d) no-one can say as the duration is very variable and depends on many factors.

4 Which of the following is the best advice to give Mr Aghomi when he asks 'What can my wife have to eat?' Give her:
   (a) a low-protein diet and plenty of glucose drinks for the first few days,
   (b) a high-protein and high-carbohydrate intake to aid the return of liver function,
   (c) only glucose drinks for the first few days,
   (d) a high-protein but low-fat diet initially.

5 Which of the following is the correct explanation to give if Mrs Aghomi asks 'Am I infectious?'
   (a) the disease was infectious before the jaundice became noticeable,
   (b) yes, you are but your family will be given vaccinations,
   (c) only the blood taken for various investigations is likely to transmit the infection,
   (d) we will give you some globulin to combat the disease and prevent you being infectious.

6 Which one of the following may occur if Mrs Aghomi did not obey her general practitioner's advice about rest? She could:
   (a) cause a persistence of the hepatitis into a chronic phase,
   (b) suffer from posthepatitis syndrome,
   (c) develop acute hepatic necrosis,
   (d) precipitate aplastic anaemia.

7 Which one of the following instructions should Mrs Aghomi be given as she is beginning to recover?
   (a) continue a low-fat diet,
   (b) abstain from alcohol for at least 3 months,
   (c) convalesce for 4 weeks before returning to work,
   (d) try to achieve her ideal weight to improve her recovery.

ANSWERS TO EXAMPLE

Mrs Funmi Aghomi

1 (c) Only correct answer.

2 (a) Rest is important and added energy expenditure will prolong the time necessary for the liver to recover.

3 (b) Jaundice is a variable feature of hepatitis but tends to occur as the most acute phase is ending before recovery.

4 (d) Bile production so necessary to fat digestion is impaired and ingestion of fats will induce nausea.

5 (a) True. People are infectious when suffering from hepatitis even though they may not experience obvious jaundice.

6 (c) The liver has great powers of healing and regeneration but rest is essential to aid the process.

7 (b) Detoxification of 'poison' such as alcohol is an ability which is delayed during liver recovery.

Mr Richard Brook,   a 52-year-old accountant, is admitted to your ward for pre-operative preparation before undergoing an abdomino-perineal excision of rectum.

1 Which one of the following is considered to be associated with carcinoma of the rectum?
   (a) high saturated-fat intake,
   (b) regular aperients,
   (c) regional enteritis,
   (d) low-fibre diets.

2 Which one of the following is Mr Brook most likely to have experienced?
   (a) pain and blood on defaecation,
   (b) abdominal pain and rectal bleeding,
   (c) frequent diarrhoea with blood and mucous,
   (d) alternating diarrhoea and constipation with rectal bleeding.

3 Which one of the following investigations will have confirmed Mr Brook's diagnosis? A:
   (a) sigmoidoscopy and biopsy,
   (b) barium meal and follow through,
   (c) proctoscopy and mucosal aspiration,
   (d) rectal examination and stool culture.

4 Which of the following is the most likely bowel preparation for Mr Brook? He will have:
   (a) two Beogex suppositories,
   (b) no specific preparation,
   (c) colonic irrigation,
   (d) Milpar twice daily.

5 Which one of the following is most helpful in enabling Mr Brook to accept his forthcoming colostomy?
   (a) advice from the Colostomy Association and relevant literature,
   (b) a discussion with the doctor of what the operation entails,
   (c) an assurance of adequate nursing support postoperatively,
   (d) time and opportunity to be able to express his concerns.

Mrs Diane Gibbs   is a 48-year-old lady who has been admitted to hospital after a sudden large haematemesis at home. She is accompanied by her husband.

1 Which of the following actions should be taken first when Mrs Gibbs vomits more blood on arriving in the accident and emergency department?
   (a) provide a receiver and tissues,
   (b) turn her into the semi-prone position,
   (c) call the doctor and prepare an infusion trolley,
   (d) pass a nasogastric tube and aspirate stomach contents.

2 Which of the following are symptomatic of severe blood loss?
   (a) pallor and dyspnoea,
   (b) clammy skin and tachycardia,
   (c) bradycardia and hypercapnoea,
   (d) atrial fibrillation and hypotension.

3 Which one of the following answers should the nurse give to a junior nurse who wishes to know 'What will happen to Mrs Gibbs?' She will:
   (a) be given a sedative and then go to theatre,
   (b) receive a blood transfusion and remain on bed rest,
   (c) have a nasogastric tube passed and be observed for 24 hours,
   (d) be given supportive care until her condition stabilises and the cause of the bleeding can be established.

4 Which one of the following is the reason for malignant ulcers bleeding profusely?
   (a) they grow rapidly,
   (b) they are more vascular than benign ulcers,
   (c) thrombocytes are reduced in malignant disease,
   (d) afibrinogenaemia develops due to the malignancy.

5 Which one of the following is true of malignant gastric ulcers? Recent medical evidence now shows that:
   (a) they start as malignant ulcers,
   (b) they develop from benign ulcers,
   (c) the associated pain is due to pancreatic invasion,
   (d) they are more commonly associated with hyperchlorhydria.

6 Which one of the following drugs is most effective in reducing bleeding from a malignant gastric ulcer?
   (a) diazepam,
   (b) vitamin K,
   (c) morphine sulphate,
   (d) propantheline bromide.

Mr Albert Haines, aged 45 years, works for a large removal firm. He is admitted to the accident and emergency department with a suspected strangulated inguinal hernia.

1 Which one of the following best describes an inguinal hernia? It is due to a weakness in the:
   (a) groin where the femoral artery emerges,
   (b) extraperitoneal intra-abdominal fascia,
   (c) abdominal wall where the spermatic cord emerges,
   (d) abdominal wall due to straining of the rectus abdominis.

2 Which one of the following best describes a strangulated inguinal hernia? It is that:
   (a) the bowel has twisted on itself,
   (b) the hernia cannot be reduced manually,
   (c) the blood supply has become cut off,
   (d) restricting adhesions of the bowel have occurred.

3 With which of the following symptoms is Mr Haines most likely to present?
   (a) vomiting, pain and pyrexia,
   (b) pyrexia, pain and constipation,
   (c) constipation and difficulty in passing urine,
   (d) increased peristalsis, vomiting and diarrhoea.

4 For which of the following should the nurses perpare Mr Haines?
   (a) bowel decompression,
   (b) pre-operative catheterisation,
   (c) intravenous fluids to correct electrolyte imbalance,
   (d) intravenous fluids and the passing of a nasogastric tube.

5 Which one of the following is most likely to occur if Mr Haines is not operated on immediately?
   (a) chronic obstruction,
   (b) general peritonitis,
   (c) gangrenous intestine,
   (d) mesenteric adenitis.

6 Which one of the following is the most likely complication that Mr Haines may develop after his operation?
   (a) impotence,
   (b) varicocoel,
   (c) epididymo-orchitis,
   (d) premature ejaculation.

Kevin Jones   is 10 weeks old and was born with a cleft lip and palate. He is admitted to the paediatric ward for repair of the cleft lip and his mother is to stay with him.

1 Which one of the following is the reason for performing this operation so soon after birth?
(a) it is before teething begins,
(b) the operation will be less painful,
(c) it is before further facial development,
(d) it will be easier to re-establish feeding.

2 Which one of the following is the major problem regarding Kevin's care? He:
(a) has difficulty in feeding,
(b) cannot retain his feeds,
(c) is more prone to infection,
(d) has difficulty in gaining weight.

3 Which of the following is the most important aspect of Kevin's specific pre-operative care?
(a) ensuring Mrs Jones continues to breast feed,
(b) feeding him with a spoon and giving water after feeds,
(c) passing a nasogastric tube and instituting gastric feeds,
(d) give no feeds to Kevin for at least 6 hours before operation.

4 Which one of the following is the most significant postoperative observation for the nurse to make on Kevin?
(a) pulse rate,
(b) temperature,
(c) fluid intake,
(d) respiration rate.

5 Which one of the following is the most effective way of preventing Kevin from touching his lip?
(a) apply elbow splints,
(b) wrap him in a blanket,
(c) let his mother hold him,
(d) lie him in the prone position.

James Kent is a 27-year-old taxi driver who has been admitted to your ward for excision of recurrent pilonidal sinus.

1 Which of the following best describes Mr Kent's pilonidal sinus? It is a:
   (a) sclerosis of sacral veins causing inadequate venous drainage,
   (b) pathway through an infected muscle sheath at the base of the spine,
   (c) focus of infection resulting from ingrowing body hairs,
   (d) purulent sacral wound derived from an anal fistula.

2 Which one of the following should minimise the possibility of Mr Kent developing postoperative wound infection?
   (a) pre-operative bowel cleansing by enema,
   (b) skin shaving and application of iodine,
   (c) maintaining a supine position when in bed,
   (d) Savlon baths twice daily and on the morning of surgery.

3 In which of the following positions should Mr Kent be nursed post-operatively?
   (a) left lateral to enhance drainage,
   (b) prone, to facilitate wound healing,
   (c) semi-recumbent, to maintain even pressure,
   (d) orthopnoeic, to shift pressure from sacrum to ischium.

4 Which one of the following replies should you give to Mr Kent when he asks would fibre in his diet reduce the chances of a further recurrence?
   (a) no, because the pattern of your pilonidal sinus is already established,
   (b) yes, because efficient bowel function resists the formation of sinuses,
   (c) no, because your disorder is not connected with your diet as far as it is known,
   (d) yes, but only if you are prepared to adhere to a strict regimen.

5 Which of the following best explains marsupialisation to the junior nurse who wishes to understand the surgery performed on Mr Kent? It involves excision of infected tissue and:
   (a) formation of pouch from the skin ends,
   (b) a division of the muscle and skin layers,

(c) approximation of the skin edges to prevent rechannelling,

(d) insertion of purse string sutures surrounding the area of repair.

6 Which of the following advice should you give Mr Kent before his discharge home?

(a) bath at least once a day,

(b) avoid straining to defaecate,

(c) try to adopt a sleeping position which keeps you off your buttocks,

(d) change your job to one which does not involve sitting down.

7 Which one of the following statements is true of Mr Kent's pilonidal sinus? It is:

(a) easily acquired by dark-skinned people,

(b) an hereditary disorder,

(c) potentially malignant,

(d) predominant in males.

Mr John Blowes,   aged 68 years, has been discharged home for terminal care following the recurrence of a carcinoma of the large bowel, after a previous left hemicolectomy, and the discovery of extensive metastases. Mrs Blowes has osteoarthritis of both knees.

1 Which of the following services are the most appropriate to help this couple to maintain their independence?
   (a) meals on wheels, domiciliary physiotherapy and district nursing,
   (b) meals on wheels, home help and district nursing,
   (c) home help, social services and health visiting,
   (d) home help, laundry service and meals on wheels.

2 Which of the following is the best reason for Mr Blowes being asked to keep a pain chart? To assess the:
   (a) risk of drug overdosage,
   (b) development of addiction,
   (c) effectiveness of his analgesia,
   (d) time at which his pain is least.

3 Which of the following is the most appropriate measure to relieve Mr Blowes' constipation?
   (a) an enema twice a week,
   (b) paraffin emulsion twice daily,
   (c) glycerine suppositories nightly,
   (d) increased helpings of green vegetables at lunch time.

4 Which of the following nursing measures should provide a temporary solution to Mr Blowes' nausea? Suggest that he:
   (a) tries to eat more regularly,
   (b) takes fluids only for today,
   (c) eats only dry toast,
   (d) takes deep breaths.

5 Which of the following should help to relieve Mr Blowes' anxiety about disturbing his wife when he is restless during the night? Advise him to discuss with his wife whether:
   (a) he should sleep in an adjoining room,
   (b) she is disturbed by his restlessness,
   (c) he should ask the doctor for some sleeping tablets,
   (d) he should ask to have his strong analgesic mixture increased at night.

6 Which of the following actions should Mrs Blowes be advised to take if her husband's condition suddenly deteriorates?
   (a) call the district nurse,
   (b) telephone the hospital,
   (c) request an ambulance,
   (d) send for the general practitioner.

Mrs Mabel Clark,   aged 42 years, is a schoolteacher and has been feeling unwell for some weeks. She has already had several attacks of severe abdominal pain and has been admitted to hospital with suspected biliary colic. On admission the nurse noted that Mrs Clark appeared to be jaundiced.

1 Which of the following should the nurse expect Mrs Clark to be excreting?
(a) pale colourless urine,
(b) clay-coloured faeces,
(c) scanty yellow urine,
(d) dark faeces.

2 For which of the following reasons is Mrs Clark given a 'fatty meal' during her cholecystogram? It demonstrates the ability of the sphincter of Oddi to:
(a) relax and the gall bladder to relax,
(b) relax and the gall bladder to contract,
(c) contract and the gall bladder to relax,
(d) contract and the gall bladder to contract.

3 For which of the following reasons is Mrs Clark likely to have an intravenous cholangiogram rather than a cholecystogram? If:
(a) she has surgery it is performed to make sure the common bile duct is free of stones,
(b) a T-tube has been inserted as part of the operative procedure,
(c) the gall bladder does not show up with oral contrast media,
(d) the serum bilirubin is raised above normal values.

4 For which of the following reasons is vitamin K prescribed for Mrs Clark before her surgery? It:
(a) prevents jaundice from increasing,
(b) prevents deep vein thrombosis,
(c) minimises fibrinogenaemia,
(d) improves clot formation.

5 Which one of the following actions should be taken if the theatre porter arrives to collect Mrs Clark before she has received her premedication?
(a) give the premedication immediately,
(b) ask the porters to return in 30 minutes,

(c) ring the theatre sister and ask for the list to be changed,
(d) send the patient and notify the anaesthetist that no pre-medication has been given.

6 Which of the following occurs after cholecystectomy and exploration of the common bile duct?
(a) the liver takes over the function of the gall bladder,
(b) bile is no longer available for fat emulsification,
(c) bile is excreted in larger amounts in the urine,
(d) bile is stored in the common bile duct.

7 Which of the following is the reason for Mrs Clark having a T-tube present after her cholecystectomy and exploration of the common bile duct? It:
(a) allows bile to bypass the healing bile duct,
(b) is needed for a postoperative cholangiogram,
(c) allows for accurate measurement of bile production per 24 hours,
(d) acts as a safety valve in case a stone is still present in the bile duct.

Mr Paul Oliver, a 56-year-old publican, had been feeling unwell for some time and he visited his general practitioner for a check up. On examination it was noted that he had swollen ankles, splenomegaly and gynaecomastia (all suggestive of cirrhosis of the liver). Mr Oliver's admission to hospital was arranged for further investigation and treatment.

1 Which of the following is the best explanation of the term cirrhosis of the liver to give a third-year student nurse? It is:
   (a) fibrosis of the liver parenchyma,
   (b) a chronic liver disease with many causes,
   (c) variable liver cell damage accompanied by fibrosis and formation of regeneration nodules,
   (d) patchy necrosis maximal in the centrilobular zones with an associated cholestasis and cholangitis.

2 Which of the following explanations is the best one to give a student nurse who asks 'Why does Mr Oliver have ankle oedema and ascites?' It is due to:
   (a) portal hypertension changing the normal tissue fluid drainage of the area,
   (b) the liver being unable to produce sufficient plasma proteins as well as retention of salt and water from secondary hyperaldosteronism,
   (c) obstruction of blood flow through the liver and the opening up of portal systemic collaterals,
   (d) poisoning of renal function by the products of bacterial breakdown of protein that are not detoxified by the damaged liver.

3 Which of the following signs and symptoms should indicate to the nurse that Mr Oliver is on the verge of hepatic coma?
   (a) intention tremor of the hands, halitosis and aggression,
   (b) erythematous palms, ecchymoses and increasing girth,
   (c) flapping tremor of the hands, confusion and stupor,
   (d) haematemesis, jaundice and glycosuria.

4 Which one of the following dietary regimens should be adopted if Mr Oliver shows signs of impending hepatic coma? Protein should be:
   (a) restricted to less than 40g daily,
   (b) increased in amount to aid hepatic recovery,
   (c) eliminated from his diet until his condition improves,

(d) balanced according to fat and carbohydrate intake and his metabolic rate.

5 Which of the following additional measures are most likely to be included in Mr Oliver's management?
(a) 4-hourly blood pressure recordings and blood transfusions,
(b) daily urinalysis and paracentesis abdominis,
(c) an increased calorie intake and diuretics,
(d) daily girth measurements and antibiotics.

6 Which of the following observations means that further change in Mr Oliver's dietary management is required? He has:
(a) pale stools and a raised blood pressure,
(b) indigestion and is putting on weight,
(c) increasing oedema and is confused,
(d) nausea and halitosis.

7 Which of the following should the nurse expect if Mr Oliver has a Sengstaken tube inserted for bleeding oesophageal varices? He:
(a) cannot take anything by mouth or even swallow his saliva,
(b) will be in danger of disturbing the tube and so a semi-recumbent position is essential,
(c) will need frequent gastric aspiration to remove blood from the stomach,
(d) must have the balloon released for 1 minute every hour to prevent pressure necrosis of the oesophagus.

8 Which of the following is the most important measure in preventing Mr Oliver's mouth from becoming dry and dirty?
(a) 4-hourly mouthwashes of glycerine and thymol,
(b) maintenance of adequate hydration,
(c) use of salivary stimulants,
(d) ice to suck every hour.

Mrs Sarah Redford, aged 33 years, was widowed 6 months ago. She complained of 'heartburn' and difficulty in swallowing. She attended the out-patient department and subsequently was diagnosed as having achalasia.

1 Which one of the following is the best explanation of this condition to the junior nurse in the out-patient department? It is:
   (a) spasm of the lower third of the oesophagus,
   (b) benign ulceration of the oesophageal sphincter,
   (c) a reflux of gastric juice into the lower end of the oesophagus,
   (d) a protrusion of the upper end of the stomach into the oesophagus.

2 Which of the following investigations should be performed to confirm Mrs Redford's diagnosis?
   (a) oesophageal pressure measurements,
   (b) barium meal and follow through,
   (c) barium swallow,
   (d) gastroscopy.

3 Which of the following is the best advice to offer Mrs Redford regarding her eating habits.
   (a) eat small amounts of food and follow with iced soda water,
   (b) avoid alcohol and very hot or very cold food,
   (c) eat slowly and sit up straight when eating,
   (d) eat only warm food and lay down after meals.

4 Which of the following types of drugs are absolutely contraindicated for Mrs Redford?
   (a) anticholinergic agents, e.g. propantheline bromide,
   (b) corticosteroids, e.g. prednisolone,
   (c) anticoagulants, e.g. phenindione,
   (d) beta blockers, e.g. propranolol.

5 Which of the following is the best advice to give Mrs Redford when she says 'How am I supposed to manage when I am invited out?' Advise her to:
   (a) only invite people to her own home,
   (b) refuse all invitations for the time being,
   (c) try to eat in places where she can stand up and eat,
   (d) explain her difficulties when accepting the invitation.

6 Which of the following is the most usual treatment to try first for this condition?
    (a) division of muscular fibres encircling the narrowed oesophagus to allow protrusion of the mucosa,
    (b) division of the muscular fibres at the cardiac end of the stomach to relieve the stricture,
    (c) pneumatic dilation of the lower end of the oesophagus,
    (d) anastomosis of the oesophagus on to the stomach to form a new sphincter.

Emily Wood   is the 6-week-old baby daughter of Peter and Anne. Despite a good appetite Emily is not putting on weight and the health visitor has asked the local general practitioner to examine her as she suspects Emily may have fibrocystic disease of the pancreas.

1 Which one of the following is true of fibrocystic disease? It is a disease which is:
(a) familial,
(b) inherited,
(c) congenital,
(d) iatrogenic.

2 Which of the following are most indicative of fibrocystic disease?
(a) viscid mucus, retention of secretions, secondary infection and fibrosis,
(b) failure to thrive, rectal prolapse and sodium excretion from sweat glands,
(c) primary biliary cirrhosis, diarrhoea and repeated chest infections,
(d) bile duct obstruction, portal hypertension, intestinal distension and bronchiectasis.

3 Which one of the following is the simplest diagnostic test for fibrocystic disease for Emily?
(a) histological examination of the jejunal mucosa,
(b) measurement of sweat concentration,
(c) pancreatic-function tests,
(d) faecal fat estimation.

4 Which of the following is the single most important factor in Emily's treatment?
(a) effective treatment of respiratory disease,
(b) provision of salt supplements,
(c) administration of pancreatin,
(d) a low-fat diet.

5 Which of the following techniques will Anne and Peter have to learn in order to care for Emily effectively?
(a) administration of aerosol chemotherapy,
(b) postural coughing and percussion,

(c) administration of pancreatin,

(d) tube feeding.

6 Which of the following special preventive measures should Emily receive?

(a) sleep in a mist tent at night,

(b) isolation in a plastic 'bubble',

(c) passive exercises night and morning,

(d) vaccination for measles, pertussis and influenza.

7 Which of the following answers should the nurse give if Mrs Wood asks 'Is the disease fatal?'

(a) not these days as modern treatment is so much improved,

(b) with prompt treatment the greater majority of patients reach adolescence,

(c) I'm afraid most children die in their first year,

(d) only if the disease is left untreated.

8 Which of the following is the best advice for the nurse to give if Mr Wood asks 'Should we have any more children?'

(a) would you like to discuss it with sister,

(b) this is something you should discuss with your general practitioner,

(c) I will make an appointment for you both to see a genetic counsellor so that you can discuss it fully,

(d) I cannot answer your question, you must ask the consultant paediatrician.

Mrs Hilda Jupp,   a widow aged 61 years, is very obese (119kg). She has visited her general practitioner with symptoms suggestive of hiatus hernia and he arranged an out-patient appointment with a view to further investigations.

1 Which of the following is the most common manifestation of oesophageal reflux?
(a) heartburn,
(b) dysphagia,
(c) flatulence at night,
(d) regurgitation of food.

2 Which one of the following explanations should be given to Mrs Jupp to prepare her for a barium meal?
(a) a series of X-rays will be required so the procedure may take the whole morning,
(b) you must have someone to accompany you home after the X-ray,
(c) the test is painless and takes about 30 minutes,
(d) you will have to fast the day before the X-ray.

3 Which one of the following is the specific aim of asking Mrs Jupp to lose weight? To:
(a) increase the effectiveness of gastric emptying,
(b) decrease venous stasis,
(c) increase gastric motility,
(d) reduce intra-abdominal pressure.

4 Which of the following dietary advice should Mrs Jupp be given?
(a) drink plenty of milk,
(b) eat foods high in fibre,
(c) take small meals regularly, within your calorie limit,
(d) eat easily digestible and pureed foods only.

5 Which of the following should best help Mrs Jupp reduce her oesophageal reflux?
(a) lie down for 30 minutes after a meal,
(b) avoid activities that involve stooping,
(c) sleep with the foot of the bed elevated,
(d) avoid chairs with little back support.

6 For which of the following reasons should Mrs Jupp's dietician only allow a small fat intake per day? Fatty foods:
   (a) may cause nausea,
   (b) increase pylorospasm,
   (c) delay gastric emptying,
   (d) increase gastric secretions.

7 Which one of the following is a common complication of hiatus hernia?
   (a) anaemia,
   (b) dyspnoea,
   (c) achalasia,
   (d) supervening gastric carcinoma.

Mr John Belling   is a 48-year-old man who has been admitted to your ward with a confirmed diagnosis of acute infective hepatitis.

1 Which one of the following incubation periods has infective hepatitis?
   (a) 0-5 days,
   (b) 9-14 days,
   (c) 15-50 days,
   (d) 51-150 days.

2 Which one of the following is the reason for Mr Belling's nausea?
   (a) fat accumulation,
   (b) bilirubin retention,
   (c) inadequate bile excretion,
   (d) inadequate bile production.

3 Which one of the following manifestations is usual with infective hepatitis? A distaste for:
   (a) cigarettes,
   (b) alcohol,
   (c) fish,
   (d) meat.

4 Which one of the following should be reduced in the diet?
   (a) glucose,
   (b) thiamine,
   (c) protein,
   (d) potassium.

5 Which one of the following should be prescribed for Mr Belling?
  (a) total bed rest,
  (b) nursed in isolation,
  (c) up for toilet purposes,
  (d) reverse barrier nursing.

6 Which one of the following preventive measures should be encour-
  aged in the future for Mr Belling?
  (a) thorough cooking of food,
  (b) gamma-globulin when at risk,
  (c) drink mineral waters only when abroad,
  (d) careful hand washing after defaecation.

Mr John Finch, a 52-year-old married journalist, has just had an abdomino-perineal excision of rectum for carcinoma of the rectum.

1 In which of the following positions should Mr Finch be nursed on regaining consciousness?
   (a) semi-prone,
   (b) sitting upright,
   (c) on alternate sides,
   (d) with two pillows only.

2 Which one of the following indicates that peristalsis has returned?
   (a) flatus is in the colostomy bag,
   (b) he has the desire to open his bowels,
   (c) mucus is discharged from the stomal orifice,
   (d) nothing further is aspirated from the nasogastric tube.

3 Which one of the following is the reason for Mr Finch having an indwelling urethral catheter postoperatively?
   (a) he may be incontinent of urine after his operation,
   (b) there is a danger the ureters may have been damaged,
   (c) to enable an accurate output of urine to be recorded,
   (d) the bladder is in close proximity to the area of excision.

4 Which of the following is the main aim of Mr Finch's plan for discharge? He:
   (a) knows he can ring the ward should he feel he cannot manage,
   (b) has been visited by a member of the Colostomy Association,
   (c) feels confident in his ability to manage his colostomy,
   (d) has been visited by the stoma therapist.

5 Which of the following is the most important in caring for the skin around Mr Finch's stoma?
   (a) the area should be kept clean and dry,
   (b) a cream with a paraffin base should be applied to the area,
   (c) the bag should be changed immediately after the colostomy works,
   (d) any oozing from the abdominal wound should not contaminate the skin.

6 Which one of the following foods may be recommended to Mr Finch to reduce faecal odour?
   (a) yoghurt,

(b) cheese,

(c) cream,

(d) eggs.

7 Which of the following is the best advice to give Mr Finch about his diet?

(a) eat plenty of fresh fruit and vegetables so that the colostomy works regularly,

(b) take vitamin supplements as these will not now be absorbed by the intestine,

(c) he should be able to eat a normal diet like anyone else,

(d) trial and error will indicate which foods to avoid.

8 Which one of the following answers should you give Mr Finch in response to him asking about resuming sexual relations with his wife?

(a) you may have some difficulty initially,

(b) impotence is very common after this type of surgery,

(c) you should have no problems once the perineal wound has healed,

(d) I will make an appointment for you to see the psychosexual counsellor.

Mrs Hale is a 64-year-old woman who has been to theatre for surgical removal of a gastric ulcer. During surgery the ulcer was seen to be malignant and a total gastrectomy and oesophago-jejunal anastomosis was performed.

1 Which one of the following should you reply when a junior nurse asks, 'When will the nasogastric tube be removed?'
   (a) when fluids are tolerated,
   (b) as soon as bowel sounds return,
   (c) when interim suture healing is assured,
   (d) as soon as the aspirate is no longer blood stained.

2 Which of the following should cause you to suspect leakage from Mrs Hale's anastomosis? She has:
   (a) vomiting and weight loss,
   (b) weight loss and diarrhoea,
   (c) diarrhoea and abdominal pain,
   (d) abdominal pain and raised temperature.

3 Which one of the following should cause the nurse to suspect an obstruction has occurred at Mrs Hale's operation site some 3 days postoperatively? There is:
   (a) increased aspirate,
   (b) regurgitation,
   (c) constipation,
   (d) pain.

4 Which one of the following should prevent infection of Mrs Hale's thoraco-abdominal wound?
   (a) daily dressings,
   (b) daily inspection and redressing,
   (c) retain occlusive dressing until sutures are removed,
   (d) apply a sterile pad to cover the dressing when oozing occurs.

5 Which one of the following should be adopted as the best way of informing Mrs Hale that her stomach ulcer was malignant?
   (a) allow the nurse who has formed a close relation with her to be present when you tell her,
   (b) act upon the group decision made by the health-care team who know her best,
   (c) delay giving information until advice is received from the family,
   (d) wait until she asks.

Miss Janet Gray,   aged 32 years, is admitted to the ward with a diagnosis of ulcerative colitis. She has been very tired for several weeks and said she had lost weight. She complained of diarrhoea and had noticed blood in her stools. She was reluctant to go to her general practitioner as she lives with and cares for her elderly parents.

1 Which of the following is the most likely cause of Janet's tiredness?
   (a) eating a special diet,
   (b) having diarrhoea at night,
   (c) losing blood in her stools,
   (d) excessive loss of fluids and electrolytes.

2 Which of the following explanations should Janet be given in preparation for colonoscopy?
   (a) a small telescope is used to examine your large bowel,
   (b) this is a simple routine investigation so there is no need to worry,
   (c) there is no special preparation, the nurse will fetch you when the doctor is ready,
   (d) you will have an intravenous injection which means you will not know anything about it.

3 Which of the following will help Janet to cope with the embarrassment of her diarrhoea?
   (a) allocate her to a single room,
   (b) talk to the other patients and explain,
   (c) allocate her to a bed near the lavatories,
   (d) give her a can of air freshener to keep in her locker.

4 Which of the following arrangements is most important for the nurse to make with regard to Janet and her parents while she is in hospital? Request the:
   (a) neighbour to call in twice a day,
   (b) district nurse to call in and see them,
   (c) health visitor to put them on her visiting list,
   (d) social services to arrange meals on wheels and a home help.

5 For which of the following might Janet require emergency surgery?
   (a) toxic dilation of the colon,
   (b) erosion of the intestinal mucosa,
   (c) bleeding due to vitamin B deficiency,
   (d) development of malignant changes in the colon.

Mrs Hamlyn   is a 54-year-old lady who has been admitted to your ward following an attack of acute cholecystitis. She is slightly jaundiced, feels sick and complains of abdominal tenderness. Her skin feels itchy and her temperature is raised.

1 Which one of the following is the reason for Mrs Hamlyn's jaundiced skin?
   (a) an over-production of bile pigment,
   (b) an accumulation of bilirubin in the blood,
   (c) failure to excrete stercobilin from the bowel,
   (d) inappropriate renal excretion of urobilinogen.

2 Which one of the following is the reason for Mrs Hamlyn's pruritus? The:
   (a) decreased bile flow,
   (b) excretion of soluble bilirubin,
   (c) retention of circulating bile salts,
   (d) insolubility of plasma-bound bilirubin.

3 Which one of the following should relieve Mrs Hamlyn's discomfort from pruritus?
   (a) saline baths as required,
   (b) twice daily emolient baths,
   (c) applications of antihistamine cream,
   (d) frequent applications of calamine lotion.

4 Which one of the following is the likely cause of Mrs Hamlyn's cholecystitis?
(a) hepatic parenchymatous disease,
(b) biliary insufficiency,
(c) hepatic obstruction,
(d) cholelithiasis.

5 For which of the following treatments should Mrs Hamlyn be
prepared?
(a) bed rest and fluids only,
(b) choledocholithotomy and low-fat diet,
(c) bed rest, antibiotics and analgesia,
(d) cholecystostomy and reducing diet.

Mrs Rose Jackson   is 58 years old and has advanced carcinoma of the stomach. She has been admitted to the ward for terminal care as she lives alone. Mrs Jackson was widowed 3 years ago when her husband died of carcinoma of bronchus. She has a married daughter, Janice, who works full-time as a personal secretary to a business manager. She and her husband are buying and furnishing their home. Janice's brother Tom has emigrated to Canada.

1 Which one of the following will be the best reply when Mrs Jackson says to the nurse 'I am sure I caught cancer from my husband. Do you think I may have given it to my daughter?'
   (a) no, of course not, it is not catching,
   (b) it is possible but nobody knows the cause of cancer yet,
   (c) I can't tell you, as research is going on at present to try to find the cause,
   (d) it is most unlikely but the cause of cancer is not yet proven.

2 Which of the following courses of action should be taken by the nurse when Janice visits her mother and complains that she appears untidy?
   (a) ask her to put her complaint in writing so that the nursing officer can deal with it,
   (b) explain that the ward is exceptionally busy today but you will pass on her complaint to sister,
   (c) show Janice the care plan and explain the aim of the planned personal programme,
   (d) say that her mother is restless and soon looks untidy and ask if she would like to help by washing her mother's hands and face.

3 Which one of the following is most likely to be the reason for Janice's complaint?
   (a) she feels that she should be looking after her mother herself,
   (b) she thinks that her mother will get more attention if she makes a fuss,
   (c) Mrs Jackson's care has been allocated to a junior nurse,
   (d) the nursing care has been very poorly planned.

4 Which of the following actions should the night nurse take when Tom arrives $1\frac{1}{2}$ hours after his mother's death?

  (a) tell him he is unfortunately too late to see his mother alive,
  (b) give him a cup of tea in Sister's office while he waits for the doctor to arrive,
  (c) explain that his mother has died and ask if he would like to see her,
  (d) tell him you are very sorry but she has only been dead a few minutes and there was nothing he could have done.

Mr Brian Jefferson,   aged 29 years, has been admitted to hospital for removal of a salivary gland calculus after a sialogram of the submandibular glands.

1 Which of the following is the best explanation of a sialogram to give Mr Jefferson? It is:
   (a) an X-ray taken with a special machine that produces a computer printout,
   (b) an X-ray in which a minute quantity of dye is injected into the duct of the salivary gland,
   (c) a recording of the electrical activity of the vagus nerve supply to the salivary glands,
   (d) an attempt to check the size of the calculus using a lachrymal probe and X-ray.

2 For which of the following reasons do calculi more commonly occur in the submandibular glands?
   (a) the parotid duct runs a tortuous course,
   (b) their secretion is rather thick and contains mucus,
   (c) the submandibular duct is straight and secretions can accumulate,
   (d) these are the largest glands and have to produce the most secretion.

3 Which of the following is Mr Jefferson most likely to experience?
  (a) pain in the region of the facial nerve,
  (b) a dry mouth, fissured tongue and difficulty in swallowing,
  (c) a swelling that appears between meals and diminishes after eating,
  (d) a swelling that appears at meal times and diminishes in size between meals.

4 Which of the following is the best answer to give Mr Jefferson when he asks 'Why do I need an operation to remove the stone?' Because:
  (a) if left untreated an abscess may develop within the gland,
  (b) pressure on the facial nerve from the stone will cause a Bell's palsy,
  (c) any infection present can spread down into the lungs and cause pneumonia,
  (d) if the gland is damaged by repeated infections they will have to remove the glands as well as the calculus.

Mrs Edna Dawson, aged 58 years, is admitted to the ward with a provisional diagnosis of diverticulitis of the large bowel.

1 Which of the following is the best explanation to give a junior nurse when she asks 'What is diverticulitis?' It is inflammation of:
   (a) multiple polypi present in the wall of the colon,
   (b) the Peyer's patches followed by fibrosis of the colon,
   (c) mucosal herniations through the weakened colonic muscle,
   (d) outpouchings of the muscularis mucosa of the colon through its weakened adventia.

2 From which of the following signs and symptoms is Mrs Dawson likely to have suffered?
   (a) blood and mucus in her stools,
   (b) an altered bowel habit and rectal bleeding,
   (c) diarrhoea, weight loss and rectal bleeding,
   (d) alternating constipation and diarrhoea accompanied by abdominal pain.

3 Which one of the following is most likely to be included in Mrs Dawson's treatment?
   (a) Dorbanex, a steroid and an analgesic,
   (b) Isogel, an antibiotic and an analgesic,
   (c) Salazopyrin, an antipyretic and an antibiotic,
   (d) prednisolone, an antispasmodic and an antidiarrhoeal.

4 Which one of the following is the most common complication of diverticulitis?
   (a) adhesions,
   (b) peritonitis,
   (c) cancerous change,
   (d) fistulae formation.

5 Which of the following is the reason for advising Mrs Dawson to take a high-fibre diet? It will:
   (a) reduce the frequency and amount of diarrhoea,
   (b) help dislodge faeces collecting in the diverticula,
   (c) encourage the formation of a normal well-formed stool,
   (d) encourage normal peristalsis, and thus reduce the intraluminal pressure.

Jason Kelly,   aged 9 months, who was born with a cleft lip and palate, is re-admitted to the paediatric ward for repair of his cleft palate.

1 Which of the following is the best advice to give Mrs Kelly regarding feeding Jason?
   (a) he can eat and drink normally,
   (b) use only soft plastic cutlery,
   (c) increase his vitamin supplements,
   (d) she should return to bottle feeding for 2 weeks.

2 Which one the following complications may Jason develop post-operatively?
   (a) difficulty with chewing,
   (b) difficulty in swallowing,
   (c) non-alignment of maxilla,
   (d) recurrent nasal infections.

3 Which one of the following is the best advice to give Mrs Kelly when Jason goes home?
(a) don't allow him to put anything in his mouth,
(b) you shouldn't have any problems after this operation,
(c) do not treat him any differently to your other children,
(d) temporary use of a dummy will help shape his hard palate.

4 Which of the following is the best advice to give Mrs Kelly regarding future pregnancies?
(a) she should consider having a sterilisation,
(b) she must seek the advice of a genetic counsellor,
(c) it is unlikely that any further children will be affected,
(d) the chance of a further son being born with the same abnormalities is high.

Mr Richard Neale,   aged 32 years, has recently returned from a holiday in Greece with his wife and two young daughters. He returned home early from work complaining of a headache, cough and feeling generally unwell. In the morning he was feverish and Mrs Neale called their general practitioner who suspected typhoid fever and arranged for Mr Neale to be admitted to hospital.

1 Which of the following answers should you give a junior student nurse when she asks 'What is typhoid fever?' It is a/an:
   (a) disease of animals spread to man by inhalation,
   (b) enteritis caused by infection with *Toxoplasma gondii,*
   (c) virus infection with a high mortality, endemic in Africa and Europe,
   (d) septicaemia originating from invasion of the small bowel by *Salmonella typhi.*

2 By which of the following is typhoid fever spread? Via:
   (a) reheated food,
   (b) contaminated water,
   (c) inhalation of droplets,
   (d) drinking unpasteurised milk.

3 From which of the following symptoms is Mr Neale likely to suffer in the second week of his illness?
   (a) rash, delirium and muscle cramps,
   (b) dehydration, stupor and hypotension,
   (c) vomiting, fever and increased salivation,
   (d) abdominal pain, distension and diarrhoea.

4 Which one of the following investigations should confirm Mr Neale's diagnosis?
   (a) the clinical picture is pathognomonic,
   (b) blood cultures at the start of his illness,
   (c) widal reaction in the first week of his illness,
   (d) isolation of the organism from guinea pig innoculation.

5 Which of the following nursing measures are an important part of Mr Neale's care?
   (a) bed rest, barrier nursing and frequent mouth care,
   (b) bed rest, reverse barrier nursing and regular mouth care,

   (c) be allowed up for the commode, barrier nursing and a high-fibre diet,

   (d) complete isolation, 'nil by mouth' and observations of blood pressure and pulse.

6 Which of the following antibiotics is most likely to be prescribed for Mr Neale?

   (a) chloroquine,

   (b) flucloxacillin,

   (c) chloramphenicol,

   (d) oxytetracycline.

7 Which of the following complications is Mr Neale most likely to develop?

   (a) acute bronchitis,

   (b) paralytic ileus,

   (c) intestinal haemorrhage,

   (d) intestinal perforation.

8 For which one of the following reasons should Mr Neale have Vi antibodies tested, if six consecutive negative stool and urine cultures have been obtained?

   (a) relapses are common in typhoid fever,

   (b) immunity after typhoid is only partial,

   (c) he may require a booster dose of TAB vaccine,

   (d) persistence of these agglutinins indicates the patient is likely to be a 'carrier'.

Mrs Amy Pope,   aged 76 years, is a rather frail lady who lives on her own since her husband died last year. Hesitantly, she revealed to the health visitor that she had a 'prolapse'. The general practitioner discovered it to be a rectal prolapse and arranged for Mrs Pope's admission to hospital.

1 With which of the following is rectal prolapse most usually associated?
   (a) ageing, weight loss and decreasing muscle tone,
   (b) infancy, obesity and excessive toilet training,
   (c) a hypertrophic, muscular pelvic floor and childbirth,
   (d) prostatism and an increase in intra-abdominal pressure from bladder distension.

2 Which of the following symptoms is Mrs Pope most likely to reveal on sympathetic questioning?
   (a) feeling of 'something coming down'
   (b) loss of continence and escape of flatus,
   (c) persistent mucous discharge and tenesmus,
   (d) feeling of discomfort and rectal bleeding.

3 By which of the following means does the insertion of a Thiersch wire prevent rectal prolapse? It:
   (a) restricts the diameter of the anus,
   (b) causes fixation of the rectal wall,
   (c) acts like a pessary and supports the anal canal,
   (d) unites the sigmoid colon and rectum more closely.

4 For which of the following reasons is Mrs Pope most likely to have a Thiersch wire inserted as opposed to Ivalon sponge?
   (a) her age makes any other treatment unsuitable,
   (b) it obviates the need for a laparotomy,
   (c) it is a more successful operation,
   (d) no anaesthetic is required.

5 Which of the following is the most likely outcome if Mrs Pope's anal suture is too tight?
   (a) circulatory collapse,
   (b) episodic diarrhoea,
   (c) constipation,
   (d) haemorrhage.

6 Which of the following is most likely to reduce Mrs Pope's embarrassment about 'her condition'?
  (a) minimise her discomfort,
  (b) be an understanding listener if she relates problems of a personal nature,
  (c) ensure and respect her privacy when attending to personal hygiene and treatments,
  (d) elicit any concerns or questions she may have and thus assure her of your understanding.

7 Which one of the following should be established before Mrs Pope's discharge home?
  (a) daily rectal sphincter dilation,
  (b) soft easily passed faeces,
  (c) daily perianal hygiene,
  (d) changed dietary habits.

8 Which of the following information is most essential for Mrs Pope to understand? She must:
  (a) avoid laxatives so that the stool is formed rather than being soft or liquid,
  (b) have daily salt baths to relieve sphincter spasm,
  (c) never allow herself to become constipated,
  (d) apply a local anaesthetic ointment daily.

Mr Greig, a 32-year-old physical education teacher, has suffered from ulcerative colitis for some 9 years. In the last 3 months his condition has deteriorated and he has had a long period of absence from school. He has been admitted for assessment with a view to total proctocolectomy and ileostomy.

1 Which of the following gives the best description of the changes which occur in ulcerative colitis?
   (a) patchy ulceration of the mucosal lining of the large bowel,
   (b) patchy ulceration and fibrosis of the colonic adventitia,
   (c) fibrosis of the muscularis mucosa of the colon,
   (d) granulation and fibrosis of the colon wall.

2 Which one of the following preparations should Mr Greig receive before his barium enema?
   (a) no specific preparation,
   (b) high colonic lavage morning and evening,
   (c) a disposable enema followed by three rectal washouts,
   (d) nothing to eat or drink for 6 hours before the X-rays.

3 Which of the following is the most important reason why surgery is being considered for Mr Greig? To:
   (a) prevent the discomfort and inconvenience of further attacks,
   (b) prevent the onset of supervening malignant change,
   (c) improve his health and social integration,
   (d) relieve his severe fatigue.

4 Which of the following dietary advice should Mr Greig be given after his operation? He needs to:
   (a) increase his daily fluid intake,
   (b) increase his dietary roughage,
   (c) limit the intake of fat,
   (d) avoid fruit juices.

5 Which of the following activities should Mr Greig be advised to avoid in future because of his ileostomy?
   (a) swimming,
   (b) fencing,
   (c) squash,
   (d) judo.

6 Which of the following is the person Mr Greig should approach for repeat prescriptions of his ileostomy appliances? The:
   (a) district nurse,
   (b) stoma therapist,
   (c) appliance officer,
   (d) general practitioner.

Daniel, aged 10 months, is the only child of Mr and Mrs Simpson and was progressing well until he commenced solid foods. Since then he seems unable to gain weight. At the paediatric clinic the consultant suspects coeliac disease.

1 Which one of the following clinical features may also be present when the doctor examines Daniel? He has:
   (a) soft, bulky, pale stools,
   (b) redcurrant jelly stools,
   (c) diarrhoea with blood and mucus,
   (d) green, hard, constipated stools.

2 Which one of the following tests would confirm the diagnosis?
   (a) proctoscopy,
   (b) colonoscopy,
   (c) small bowel biopsy,
   (d) sigmoidoscopy and biopsy.

3 Which one of the following pathological changes takes place in this condition? There is:
   (a) loss of normal villous pattern,
   (b) abnormal proliferation of Peyer's patches,
   (c) evidence of fibrotic changes in the mucosal lining,
   (d) atrophy of the muscle fibres of the intestinal wall.

4 Which one of the following is the best answer to give Mrs Simpson when she asks 'Is there anything Daniel should not eat?'
   (a) milk or eggs,
   (b) rusks or crusts,
   (c) sweets or chocolate,
   (d) peaches or strawberries.

5 Which one of the following supplements should be added to Daniel's diet?
   (a) Marmite,
   (b) Multivite,
   (c) cod liver oil,
   (d) rose hip syrup.

6 Which one of the following is the most helpful advice to give Mrs Simpson about Daniel?
   (a) make sure he eats all his food,

(b) be aware that irritability and lack of activity is part of the disease,
(c) his diet will need to be reviewed at regular intervals by the dietician,
(d) give her literature about the Coeliac Society and suggest she joins for the support it will afford her.

7 Which one of the following is the best information to give Mrs Simpson regarding Daniel's prognosis?
(a) he may grow out of the disease in a few years time,
(b) it is likely, if she has any more children, that they too may be affected,
(c) if she does not adhere strictly to the diet Daniel will have a relapse,
(d) once he has regained his weight and the symptoms have gone he can resume a normal diet.

Mr Henry Mace   is 35 years old and has been admitted to your ward with severe abdominal pain due to peritonitis.

1 Which of the following micro-organisms is most likely to be responsible for Mr Mace's infection?
   (a) *Escherichia coli,*
   (b) *Staphylococcus albus,*
   (c) *Pseudomonas aeruginosa,*
   (d) *Streptococcus pyogenes.*

2 Which of the following should you expect to observe in Mr Mace initially?
   (a) vomiting and oliguria,
   (b) pyrexia and hectic flush,
   (c) abdominal pain and vomiting,
   (d) abdominal pain and constipation.

3 Which of the following should indicate that Mr Mace is developing paralytic ileus?
   (a) increased abdominal pain,
   (b) a temporary remission of symptoms,
   (c) prolonged and intensified vomiting,
   (d) a general worsening of his condition.

4 Which one of the following changes will occur initially in Mr Mace's peritoneum?
   (a) congestion and oedema,
   (b) ischaemia and necrosis,
   (c) fibrosis and adhesions,
   (d) exudation and transudation.

5 Which one of the following should indicate to the nurse that Mr Mace is experiencing severe abdominal pain?
   (a) adoption of the fetal position,
   (b) sitting hunched with knees up,
   (c) rolling around the bed,
   (d) rigid immobility.

6 Which one of the following should relieve Mr Mace's pain most effectively?
   (a) codeine phosphate,
   (b) dihydrocodeine,
   (c) pentazocine,
   (d) pethidine.

Mrs Simpkins   is an 85-year-old widow who has been admitted to your ward in a neglected state for investigation of her chronic constipation. She no longer has her own teeth and dislikes any food which she has to chew.

1 Which of the following factors is the most likely to contribute to Mrs Simpkins constipation?
(a) inactivity,
(b) poor appetite,
(c) ill-fitting dentures,
(d) an inadequate intake of fruit and vegetables.

2 Which of the following is the most appropriate advice to give Mrs Simpkins to improve her bowel function?
(a) add bran to all meals,
(b) add bran to the breakfast,
(c) eat fresh fruit and more fluid,
(d) eat green vegetables and fruit juice.

3 Which one of the following reasons should you give to the student nurse who asks 'Why is a colonic washout necessary before a barium enema?' To:
(a) facilitate retention of the barium,
(b) be certain of good X-ray pictures of the tract,
(c) reduce chances of impaction after the investigation,
(d) minimise the chances of inappropriate shadows on the X-rays.

4 Which of the following is the most likely reason for Mrs Simpkins to accuse the nurses of not telling her what is going on?
(a) an impaired memory is a feature of the ageing process,
(b) inhibitions decrease as age increases,
(c) deficient hearing is usual in old age,
(d) advanced age alters word perception.

5 Which one of the following is true for Mrs Simpkins? She is only entitled to receive:
(a) a widow's pension,
(b) mobility allowance,
(c) a retirement pension,
(d) attendance allowance.

6 Which of the following is the most accurate guide to the reason for Mrs Simpkins' neglected state?
  (a) social worker's profile,
  (b) health visitor's report,
  (d) a nurse's admission history,
  (d) house officer's case history.

Jeremy is 3 months old and the first son of Mr and Mrs Smyth. When the health visitor called she found Jeremy had not been gaining weight and was having difficulty with his feeds. She suspects Jeremy may have congenital pyloric stenosis.

1 Which one of the following is characteristic of the disease?
  (a) cyclical vomiting,
  (b) sunken fontanelle,
  (c) projectile vomiting,
  (d) umbilical protrusion.

2 Which one of the following is the reason for Jeremy's symptoms not being apparent at birth?
  (a) he has had little in the way of food,
  (b) his stomach has not expanded properly,
  (c) there is gradual inflammation and oedema of the pylorus,
  (d) it takes a week for the stomach to fill with undigested curds.

3 Which one of the following best describes Jeremy's stools? They are:
  (a) meconium-stained and constipated,
  (b) infrequent and constipated,
  (c) frequent and bright green,
  (d) like redcurrant jelly.

4 Which one of the following should be included in Jeremy's specific pre-operative nursing care?
  (a) performing a stomach washout,
  (b) keeping an accurate record of his vomit,
  (c) ensuring he has nothing by mouth for 6 hours,
  (d) passing a nasogastric tube for aspirations each hour.

5 Which one of the following best describes the operation (Ramstedt's) which is performed for this condition? It is an/a:
  (a) antrectomy,
  (b) pyloromyotomy,
  (c) vagotomy and pyloroplasty,
  (d) anastomosis of the pylorus and the duodenum.

6 Which one of the following would be the best answer to give Mrs Smyth when she asks how soon will Jeremy be feeding normally? After:
  (a) 6 hours,

(b) 12 hours,
(c) 24 hours,
(d) 48 hours.

7 Which one of the following is the correct answer to give Mrs Smyth when she asks if Jeremy's condition is likely to re-occur?
(a) it is possible as Jeremy is so young,
(b) the surgery has corrected it permanently,
(c) there is a slight risk if scar tissue forms,
(d) it is unlikely if you follow the dietary advice you have been given.

Don Southern,   aged 35 years, married with two children, works in the sales department of a large firm. Many of his business deals take place over lunch and his work involves a lot of travelling by car. His consumption of alcohol has increased to such an extent his wife has asked him to seek medical advice. He is admitted to hospital for assessment.

1 Which of the following is the main reason for recording Mr Southern's observations frequently? He may:
  (a) have a convulsion,
  (b) develop acute liver failure,
  (c) lapse into hyperglycaemic coma,
  (d) collapse due to generalised vasoconstriction.

2 Which one of the following may be prescribed for Mr Southern to prevent withdrawal symptoms?
  (a) regular sedation,
  (b) daily anticonvulsants,
  (c) abstention from alcohol,
  (d) small amounts of alcohol.

3 Which one of the following drugs may be used if aversion therapy is considered for Mr Southern?
  (a) dimercaprol,
  (b) apomorphine,
  (c) disulfiram,
  (d) methadone.

4 Which of the following is the best description to give the nurse when she asks 'What is delirium tremens?' It is:
  (a) hallucinations and feeling of grandeur,
  (b) incidence of severe manic depression,
  (c) agitation, fear and hallucination,
  (d) loss of memory and confabulations.

5 Which of the following is the best advice to give Mrs Southern regarding her husband's diet? Give him a:
  (a) high-fibre low-fat diet,
  (b) low-protein low-fat diet,
  (c) high-protein diet with vitamin supplements,

(d) diet that avoids highly spiced food and those with a high fat content.

6 Which of the following is the best answer to Mrs Southern when she asks how she can help Don's recovery?
(a) accompany him when he goes to the pub,
(b) ring Alcoholics Anonymous if you need help,
(c) be supportive and help him to occupy his leisure hours,
(d) reduce his contact with the children as the extra stress could cause unprovoked violence.

Mrs Carol Tibbs, aged 48 years, is admitted to the ward for excision of haemorrhoids (haemorrhoidectomy).

1 Which of the following signs and symptoms is Mrs Tibbs likely to have experienced?
   (a) alternating diarrhoea and constipation,
   (b) tenesmus and blood-streaked mucus,
   (c) mucus, bleeding and diarrhoea,
   (d) pain, bleeding and pruritis.

2 Which one of the following should be given priority on Mrs Tibbs' first postoperative day?
   (a) elevation of the foot of the bed,
   (b) maintenance of adequate analgesia,
   (c) ensure the rectal pack is renewed,
   (d) observation of temperature, pulse and respiration.

3 Which one of the following long-term complications is Mrs Tibbs most likely to develop after her surgery?
   (a) anal stricture,
   (b) prolapsed rectum,
   (c) perianal haematoma,
   (d) ischiorectal abscess.

4 Which one of the following should Mrs Tibbs be given post-operatively to aid bowel action?
(a) Proctofoam,
(b) Isogel granules,
(c) paraffin emulsion,
(d) Anusol suppositories.

5 Which of the following is the best advice to give Mrs Tibbs on her discharge home?
(a) walk 2 miles a day,
(b) include more fibre in your diet,
(c) avoid sitting for long periods on cold surfaces,
(d) avoid carrying heavy weights for the next month.

Mrs Patricia Walker, aged 46 years, had celebrated her birthday with her husband at a local restaurant. By lunch time the next day she had severe abdominal pain and was vomiting. Her husband called their general practitioner who arranged Pat's admission to hospital with suspected acute pancreatitis.

1 With which of the following is acute pancreatitis most commonly associated?
   (a) alcoholism,
   (b) biliary disease,
   (c) corticosteroids,
   (d) hypercholesterolaemia.

2 Which of the following explanations should be given to Mr Walker about his wife's illness. Pancreatitis:
   (a) is a serious disorder caused essentially by the digestion of the pancreas by its own secretions,
   (b) often occurs within 12 hours after the consumption of alcohol or a large meal and is not serious,
   (c) forms a sort of cyst which contains pancreatic enzymes, fluid and blood,
   (d) is fairly common and caused by fibrotic changes around the drainage channels of the pancreas and replacement of glandular tissue.

3 Which of the following explanations should be given to Mr Walker who has come to believe that his wife's birthday treat has caused her pancreatitis?
   (a) yes, it probably did, but it could have happened to anybody,
   (b) it is likely that the meal was the final precipitating factor but not the only one,
   (c) alcohol may cause pancreatitis so it is likely that too much to drink was the cause, not the meal,
   (d) no one knows what causes pancreatitis and it is only a coincidence that she was taken ill after her birthday treat.

4 Which of the following positions should help to minimise Mrs Walker's pain while bed rest has been prescribed?
   (a) sitting upright, leaning slightly forward,
   (b) semi-recumbent with two pillows only,

(c) lying on alternate sides,
(d) lying on her right side.

5 Which of the following measures are most likely to be included in Mrs Walker's management initially?
  (a) an intravenous infusion of dextro/saline 'nil by mouth', 4-hourly morphine sulphate by injection and corticosteroids,
  (b) fluids only to drink, morphine sulphate as necessary, regular blood sugar and blood calcium levels,
  (c) 'nil by mouth', laparotomy and peritoneal toilet, antibiotics,
  (d) an intravenous infusion of normal saline, nasogastric suction, 4-hourly pethidine injections and recordings of blood pressure.

6 Which of the following nursing observations should be made to monitor Mrs Walker's progress?
  (a) accurate records of fluid intake and output, daily urinalysis and observation of stools,
  (b) frequent blood pressure recordings, 4-hourly girth measurements and daily weight,
  (c) colour of stools, urine and skin, 4-hourly temperature, blood pressure and pulse rate, daily weight,
  (d) urine volume per hour, bowel habit, daily girth measurement and fluid balance.

7 Which of the following is the correct explanation to give a junior nurse who asks about Mrs Walker's prognosis?
  (a) the prognosis depends on the severity of the attack,
  (b) the mortality rate in pancreatitis is very high because of the haemorrhage that commonly occurs as a complication,
  (c) the prognosis is poor as pancreatic abscesses often develop leading to peritonitis,
  (d) unfortunately pancreatitis often recurs as it becomes chronic and then the mortality rate gradually increases.

Mr David Tucker,   aged 52 years, has been experiencing some difficulty swallowing but ignored it until recently when his wife insisted he visit their general practitioner. Suspecting carcinoma of the oesophagus, the general practitioner has arranged Mr Tucker's urgent investigation.

1 Which of the following foods is likely to cause Mr Tucker most difficulty in swallowing?
   (a) roast potatoes,
   (b) processed peas,
   (c) fresh bread,
   (d) fried fish.

2 Which of the following is the most likely reason for Mrs Tucker insisting her husband visit the general practitioner?
   (a) Mr Tucker's voice was changing,
   (b) she noticed her husband was losing weight,
   (c) Mr Tucker was unable to conceal his distress from her,
   (d) she was concerned about the increase in her husband's drinking.

3 Which of the following is the first investigation Mr Tucker would undergo?
   (a) oesophageal aspiration and washings,
   (b) exfoliative cytology,
   (c) oesophagoscopy,
   (d) barium swallow.

4 For which of the following reasons is food and drink withheld from Mr Tucker for 4 hours after an oesophagoscopy?
   (a) there will be swelling of the oropharynx,
   (b) his swallowing reflex has not yet returned,
   (c) to limit the danger from a possible perforation,
   (d) fluids before this time will cause vomiting.

5 Which of the following best describes how neoplasia differs from all other pathological processes? It:
   (a) involves increase of the cells of the affected tissue,
   (b) may adversely affect the body's nutritional state,
   (c) is relatively independent of the body's control,
   (d) is detrimental to the host.

6 Which of the following will best minimise the risk of obstruction of the Celestin tube Mr Tucker has had inserted after his diagnosis of carcinoma of the oesophagus?
(a) a soft diet,
(b) a liquidised diet,
(c) soda water after meals,
(d) a high daily fluid intake.

7 Which of the following is the most important factor in keeping Mr Tucker's mouth clean and healthy?
(a) adequate hydration,
(b) daily oral irrigation,
(c) use of salivary stimulants,
(d) regular cleaning with mouth washes.

8 Which of the following complications will Mr Tucker develop if his oral hygiene is neglected?
(a) anorexia and peritonsillar abscess,
(b) oral 'thrush' and gastroenteritis,
(c) mouth ulcers and bronchiectasis,
(d) parotitis and gingivitis.

Mr Nigel Walsh is a 29-year-old teacher who was diagnosed as having a malabsorption syndrome, probably due to Crohn's disease, a few weeks ago. His urgent admission to hospital was arranged.

1 Which of the following is the best definition of Crohn's disease to give the junior nurse? It is a:
   (a) polyposis that affects the small bowel but occasionally affects the large bowel,
   (b) condition in which there is abnormal proliferation in the small bowel which interferes with absorption,
   (c) disease of the small bowel lining that is characterised by deformity of the normal villi,
   (d) chronic inflammatory disease of the bowel capable of attacking any part of the gut from mouth to anus.

2 From which of the following nutritional disturbances is Mr Walsh most likely to suffer?
   (a) weight loss, anaemia and hypoproteinaemia,
   (b) steatorrhoea, abdominal pain and flatulence,
   (c) watery diarrhoea, abdominal colic and tenesmus,
   (d) abdominal distension and intractable diarrhoea.

3 Which of the following investigations is most likely to be ordered for Mr Walsh to confirm the diagnosis? A:
   (a) colonoscopy,
   (b) barium enema,
   (c) sigmoidoscopy,
   (d) barium meal and follow through.

4 Which one of the following is likely to be prescribed to control Mr Walsh's diarrhoea?
   (a) codeine phosphate (15—30mg up to four times daily),
   (b) azathioprine ($2mg\ day^{-1}\ kg^{-1}$ body weight),
   (c) sulphadimidine (500mg four times daily),
   (d) sulphasalazine (1g four times daily).

5 Which of the following is the reason for prescribing bed rest for Mr Walsh initially?
   (a) it reduces his basal metabolic rate and thus reduces his oxygen debt,
   (b) he is anaemic and needs to reduce his body's demand for oxygen,

(c) rest enhances the normal healing process,
(d) it encourages erythropoiesis.

6 Which of the following is the reason that Mr Walsh is unlikely to be offered surgical treatment?
   (a) remission is common,
   (b) medical treatment is so successful,
   (c) postoperative fistulae formation are common,
   (d) surgery is dangerous after immunosuppressive therapy.

7 Which of the following dietary regimens should be recommended to Mr Walsh before his discharge home? To:
   (a) avoid vegetables with a lot of roughage and all derivatives of wheat flour,
   (b) have a low-fat diet and increase his intake of protein,
   (c) increase his intake of milk and proteins,
   (d) eat a normal diet with added vitamins.

8 Which of the following explanations is the best one to give Mr Walsh when he asks 'Why does the doctor say I must give up smoking?'
   (a) smoking increases gut movements and may make your diarrhoea worse,
   (b) smoking does cause heart disease and chronic lung disease which would add to your problems,
   (c) nicotine delays the healing process,
   (d) smoking may damage your gut lining.

Tom Wilson   is a 28-year-old batchelor working as a surveyor. For several weeks he has had pain in the anal area and after an out-patient appointment he is admitted with a diagnosis of a fistula in ano.

1 Which one of the following describes a fistula in ano? It is a:
   (a) split in the anal canal,
   (b) blind-ended track above the anal canal,
   (c) false track between the anus and the skin,
   (d) false track between the anus and the rectum.

2 Which of the following signs and symptoms is Tom most likely to have experienced?
   (a) bleeding on defaecation,
   (b) rectal bleeding of mucus and blood,
   (c) tenesmus, pain and faecal discharge,
   (d) moisture around the anus and faecal discharge.

3 Which of the following is the most likely complication if Tom's fistula remains untreated?
   (a) haemorrhoids,
   (b) rectal prolapse,
   (c) pilonidal sinus,
   (d) an anal stricture.

4 Which of the following is the most likely method of treatment for Tom's disorder?
   (a) daily packing with an Eusol wick,
   (b) daily anal dilatation and use of stool softener,
   (c) opening of the track and healing by granulation,
   (d) opening of the track and healing by first intention.

5 Which of the following is the main aim of Tom's nursing care? To:
   (a) prevent infection,
   (b) occlude the area,
   (c) monitor urinary output,
   (d) diminish anal sphincter spasm.

Mr Simon Tate   is a 52-year-old publican who has been admitted to hospital after severe bleeding from oesophageal varices. He is accompanied by his wife.

1 Which one of the following explanations should you give to a student nurse who asks 'Why do oesophageal varices occur?'
   (a) blockage of distal blood flow has occurred,
   (b) constant direct pressure impedes venous flow,
   (c) venous drainage has no gravitational support,
   (d) blood flow is impeded due to pressure changes.

2 Which one of the following is Mr Tate most likely to experience as a result of intestinal venous congestion?
   (a) diarrhoea,
   (b) flatulence,
   (c) low blood pressure,
   (d) electrolyte imbalance.

3 Which one of the following conditions leads to oesophageal varices?
   (a) cirrhosis,
   (b) carcinoid,
   (c) amyloidosis,
   (d) sarcoidosis.

4 Which one of the following explanations should be given to the student nurse who wants to know the major function of a Sengstaken tube? It:
   (a) fibroses the broken vessels,
   (b) allows for gastric aspiration,
   (c) helps to decrease the clotting time,
   (d) provides prolonged compression leading to coagulation.

5 Which one of the following dietary modifications should Mr Tate make to increase his life expectation?
   (a) high protein and increased fluids,
   (b) low protein and moderate fluids,
   (c) low fat and high protein,
   (d) low fat and low fibre.

6 Which one of the following should the nurse advise Mrs Tate who wants to help her husband? Tell her to:
   (a) ensure a diet rich in vitamin B,
   (b) encourage him to reduce his alcohol intake,
   (c) reduce the size and frequency of his meals,
   (d) encourage him to eat more slowly and follow with a rest period.

ANSWERS

Mr Richard Brook

1 (d) Low-fibre diets result in depressed bowel activity and constipation and possible carcinogens within the faeces have greater contact time with the rectal wall.
2 (d) A pathognomonic feature of carcinoma of the rectum.
3 (a) Visualisation alone is inadequate as a diagnostic measure. Confirmation requires a histological sample for analysis.
4 (c) Retrograde irrigation is essential and together with direct cleansing action ensures bowel is free from gas and faeces.
5 (d) This answer acknowledges the essential role the patient himself plays in his own recovery.

Mrs Diane Gibbs

1 (b) It is quite likely that Mrs Gibbs will lose consciousness and this position will prevent asphyxiation by vomit.
2 (b) These are the symptoms of hypovolaemia which results in an increased pulse rate, a fall in blood pressure and a redirection of blood from the periphery.
3 (d) This acknowledges that only maintenance treatment can be given until a diagnosis is made.
4 (b) Rapidly dividing cells require a good blood supply.
5 (a) Current statistical evidence supports this.
6 (c) Morphine sulphate causes constriction of the gastric blood vessels due to its effect on the autonomic nervous system.

Mr Albert Haines

1 (c) Only correct answer.
2 (c) Only correct definition.

3 (a) Vomiting due to reverse peristalsis. Pain results from attempt to overcome obstruction. Pyrexia due to inflammatory response.

4 (d) Intravenous fluids essential to correct the dehydration resulting from vomiting, sweating and extravasation of fluids in the inflammatory response. Nasogastric tube reduces the nausea/vomiting experienced from a stomach unable to empty.

5 (c) Gangrene results from an impeded blood supply due to the strangulation.

6 (c) This provides an easy route for spread of pathogenic micro-organisms from abdominal peritoneum through the inguinal canal resulting in epididymo-orchitis.

Kevin Jones

1 (c) Further facial development increases the difficulties of surgery and decreases the chances of a successful outcome.

2 (c) There is a common pathway for food and air.

3 (b) Sucking action not possible.

4 (d) An increasing respiratory rate is an early sign of respiratory obstruction.

5 (a) Effective and less likely to cause frustration for the infant.

James Kent

1 (c) Only correct definition.

2 (d) To remove as many of the surface skin bacteria as possible, without any risk of damaging the skin (i.e. by shaving).

3 (b) As a pilonidal sinus is located in the intergluteal, cleft sitting is painful after surgery and undue pressure inhibits circulation.

4 (c) There is no connection between the gut and a pilonidal sinus.

5 (c) When an abscess develops, incision and drainage is indicated and the technique is used to avoid further sinus formation.

6 (a) Reduces the risk of infection by reducing the bacterial load of the skin.

7 (d) Only correct answer, probably because men have a different amount and distribution of body hair to women.

Mr John Blowes

1 (b) The services which recognise the particular needs of Mr and Mrs Blowes.

2 (c) Ineffective analgesia is unnecessary and always to be deprecated. Raiman, J (1983) Pain, in: S Collins and E Parker (Eds) *An Introduction to Nursing*, Macmillan.

3 (a) The most appropriate measure given the patient's diagnosis.

4 (b) Fluids are essential otherwise Mr Blowes will be distressed by the effects of electrolyte imbalance and this restriction may allow the bowel time to recover.

5 (b) One must never assume levels of verbal communication which may not exist between some couples.

6 (d) Mr Blowes should be enabled to die in his own home and all efforts to remove him to hospital should be resisted.

Mrs Mabel Clark

1 (b) Bile products colour the faeces and bile is unable to enter the duodenum as the common bile duct is blocked.

2 (b) The presence of fat in the stomach causes the release of cholecystokinin (enterokinase) which relaxes the sphincter of Oddi and contracts the gall bladder.

3 (c) Only correct answer.

4 (d) Vitamin K is essential to the production of prothrombin by the liver but as it is a fat-soluble vitamin and fat is not digested due to inadequate bile levels in the duodenum during biliary obstruction it is usually deficient before surgery.

5 (d) The anaesthetist will adjust the drugs necessary to induce anaesthesia if no premedicating drug has been given.

6 (d) After cholecystectomy the common bile duct acts as a storage for bile.

7 (a) The bile duct will be oedematous (as a result of wound healing) after exploration and acts as a source of biliary obstruction until oedema subsides. Therefore bypassing is to avoid nausea and pain.

Mr Paul Oliver

1 (c) Only correct definition.

2 (b) Ascites is the result of a fall in plasma colloidal osmotic pressure due to a reduction in serum albumin. This, together with portal hypertension, leads to ascites. An increased secretion of aldosterone (possibly due to pooling of blood in the gut) promotes sodium and fluid retention.

3 (c) These are early symptoms of hepatic coma which may occur in patients with chronic liver disease and is most probably due to intoxication of the brain by products of protein digestion.

4 (a) (See also 3 above) To decrease the products of protein digestion by decreasing the amount of protein ingested should reduce symptoms.

5 (c) An increase in calories, i.e. carbohydrate will decrease breakdown of fat and protein (see 3 and 4 above). Diuretics reduce oedema and the patient often recovers physically too.

6 (c) Indicates further deterioration of liver. (See 3–5 above.)

7 (a) The inflated oesophageal balloon compresses the bleeding varices, the gastric balloon compresses the fundal veins which drain into the varices, presence of the balloons means nothing can pass down the oesophagus.

8 (b) No amount of oral toilet will keep a patient's mouth moist and clean if he is dehydrated.

Mrs Redford

1 (a) Only correct answer.

2 (c) Barium swallow often shows gross dilation of the oesophagus and barium mixing with a stagnant column of liquid which has not been emptied into the stomach from the previous meal.

3 (b) A bland diet minimises symptoms, possibly by reducing spasm.

4 (a) Anticholinergic drugs decrease oesophageal peristalsis and will worsen her symptoms.

5 (d) Having to eat slowly and chew thoroughly before swallowing can delay meals. Regurgitation is a further embarrassment.

6 (c) Dilatation obviates the need for thoracotomy, as in Heller's operation, and means a shorter stay in hospital.

Emily Wood

1 (b) Inherited as an autosomal recessive, i.e. not carried on sex

chromosome and needs gene from both mother and father to inherit.

2 (a) Characteristic of the disease.

3 (b) A basic abnormality of sodium reabsorption from the sweat glands is also found and provides a simple test for the disease.

4 (a) The viscid mucus leads to retention of secretions particularly in the lungs giving rise to bronchiectasis and emphysema if untreated.

5 (b) The treatment to prevent 4a above.

6 (d) To prevent chronic chest infections. Measles, pertussis and influenza have respiratory complications which should be avoided by vaccination.

7 (b) With the advent of effective chemotherapy 70% of patients now survive until early adulthood.

8 (c) This is the best advice to give provided there is easy access to genetic counselling!

Mrs Hilda Jupp

1 (a) This results from acid stomach contents rising into the oesophagus.

2 (c) Only correct answer.

3 (d) Loss of adipose tissue reduces the pressure against the diaphragmatic weakness and will reduce symptoms.

4 (c) Small meals will empty from the stomach more quickly and reduce discomfort.

5 (b) Avoid activities which increase the ill effects of gravity.

6 (c) The longer food remains in the stomach the greater the chance of symptoms experienced.

7 (a) Chronic blood loss from the oesophagus is the cause.

Mr John Belling

1 (c) Only correct answer.

2 (d) Inadequate bile production renders ingested fats indigestible hence nausea.

3 (a) A phenomenon without scientific explanation to date.

4 (c) The liver, which is the site of deamination (of amino acids), needs to be rested during hepatitis therefore a reduction in protein intake is required.

5 (a) Provided that total bed rest leads to a reduced body energy expenditure which is essential to liver recuperation.

6 (d) Method of spread of infective hepatitis is by the faeco-oral route, hence the need for careful handwashing.

Mr John Finch

1 (c) This avoids pressure on wound sites (both abdominal and perineal).

2 (a) Flatus which precedes faeces is a normal product of peristalsis.

3 (d) This means that interference with, and enervation of, the bladder and any resulting retention is avoided.

4 (c) This answer recognises that Mr Finch is the important person involved in his recovery.

5 (a) Essential to inhibit growth of pathogens and allow the bag to adhere to the skin properly thus avoiding soreness.

6 (a) Only correct answer.

7 (d) Much will depend on his previous dietary habits.

8 (a) The difficulties resulting from interference to innervation usually resolve, but he needs to be told the truth.

Mrs Hale

1 (b) Only correct answer.

2 (d) Pain results from chemical peritoneal irritation and a raised temperature is part of the inflammatory response.

3 (b) The nasogastric tube will have been removed so regurgitation will be suspicious of discontinuity of function of the intestine.

4 (c) This reduces the chance of introducing pathogenic micro-organisms from the exterior and allows the bactericidal properties of serum to perform without interference.

5 (d) This respects Mrs Hale's rights as an adult but does not force information on her before she is ready to receive it.

Miss Janet Gray

1 (c) Anaemia (reduction in the oxygen-carrying capacity of blood) ensures a reduced energy expenditure resulting in tiredness.

2 (a) Simple and intellectually honest.

3 (c) Urgency of defaecation necessitates use of a commode in an area

that is some distance from the toilets and embarrassment from unavoidable odour would ensue.

4 (b) The district nurse would be able to make an assessment as well as to provide care.

5 (a) This is a complication which is a surgical emergency.

Mrs Hamlyn

1 (b) Free bilirubin in the circulation, accumulating due to obstruction, results in yellow discolouration.

2 (c) Only correct answer known to date.

3 (d) Calamine lotion is a soothing agent.

4 (d) Stones are proven to be the most common cause of gall bladder infection.

5 (c) Bed rest aids the healing, antibiotics eliminate the infection and analgesics remove the pain.

Mrs Rose Jackson

1 (d) This is the most honest answer to give within our present state of knowledge.

2 (d) This answer offers to share the problem with the relative without being defensive and is likely to result in benefit to the patient.

3 (a) Guilt is experienced when we distance ourselves from sick loved ones no matter how essential it is to do so.

4 (c) The painful news has to be given and he has every right to see his mother.

Mr Brian Jefferson

1 (b) Only correct answer.

2 (b) A precipitate is more likely to form in these circumstances, as drainage is almost vertical.

3 (d) Food stimulates the production of saliva, the drainage of which is slow.

4 (a) Abscess formation is an undesirable complication of salivary gland stones.

Mrs Edna Dawson

1 (c) Only correct answer.

2 (d) These are features of diverticulitis.
3 (b) A bulking agent to stimulate the bowel, an antibiotic to eliminate the infection, an analgesic to remove the pain.
4 (b) Peritonitis is the consequence of a perforated diverticulum.
5 (d) Increased fibre stimulates peristalsis and reduces the work of colonic muscle fibres.

Jason Kelly

1 (a) This is the whole point of the surgery.
2 (d) Results from the position of the anatomical defect.
3 (c) Jason requires no special treatment.
4 (b) This is thought to be a genetically transmitted disorder.

Mr Richard Neale

1 (d) Only correct answer.
2 (b) Typhoid is spread by faeco-oral route.
3 (d) Typhoid fever is primarily a bacteraemic illness with abdominal symptoms caused by the organism invading Peyer's patches which become ulcerated.
4 (b) As already mentioned typhoid is primarily a bacteraemic illness and hence the organism can be cultured from the blood.
5 (a) Patients are extremely ill, often toxic and can become dehydrated with a foul mouth. Organisms are excreted in faeces thus barrier nursing is also required.
6 (c) The drug of choice, but not without side effects.
7 (a) An extremely common complication of typhoid, due in part to the organism's ability to lodge in the tissues as it is carried round by the blood.
8 (d) Persistence of the agglutinins indicates the patient is a 'carrier' and must take special precautions.

Mrs Amy Pope

1 (a) Only correct answer.
2 (b) As a piece of rectum prolapses through the anal canal, the anal sphincters can no longer control the passage of flatus or faeces.
3 (a) This is a non-absorbable suture inserted subcutaneously around the anus within the external sphincter layer, it only leaves a

narrow exit and thus spontaneous prolapse is less likely to occur.

4 (b) Ivalon sponge requires the insertion of plastic foam around the sigmoid colon and rectum which encourages fibrosis and fixes the rectum, but requires a laparotomy, and Mrs Pope is rather frail.

5 (c) (See 3a above) If too tight it will be difficult to pass any faeces.

6 (c) Demonstrates an awareness to the patient of your understanding and a wish to try to meet her needs.

7 (b) (See 5c) To prevent constipation.

8 (c) Constipation and straining at stool may damage the rectal mucosa with the Thiersch wire acting as a 'cheese-cutter'.

Mr Greig

1 (a) Only correct definition.

2 (a) Bowel preparation could be dangerous for this patient.

3 (b) Malignant change is common after 10 years from diagnosis.

4 (a) The operation involves removal of the large bowel and hence the area of fluid reabsorption.

5 (d) This sport is most likely to result in damage to the stoma.

6 (d) Only correct answer.

Daniel

1 (a) Due to malabsorption.

2 (c) Demonstrates that the normal villi of the small intestine are deformed or absent.

3 (a) (See 2c above) The mucosa is almost flat and thus the absorptive power is lost.

4 (b) Rusks and crusts contain gluten and in coeliac disease the mucosa is sensitive to the gliadin fraction present in gluten.

5 (b) Part of the nutritional disturbance includes vitamin deficiency hence the need to add a multivitamin preparation.

6 (d) Membership of the Coeliac Society ensures that any improvement in technique of food preparation is quickly circulated to members via news sheets.

7 (c) 'A gluten-free diet induces remission of symptoms in 80—90% of cases and it is thought that those who do not respond are not keeping to the diet.' (A.M. Dawson, St Bartholomew's Hospital, London.)

Mr Mace

1 (a) An organism normally present in the gut and likely to cause infection if it 'escapes' as in bowel perforation.

2 (c) Pain from the inflammation of the peritoneum and vomiting due to paralytic ileus, a consequence of peritonitis.

3 (b) A transient stage during which peristalsis diminishes thus causing less pain. As ileus develops effortless vomiting results and the peritonitis has progressed.

4 (a) The first signs of inflammation.

5 (d) If pain is very severe the patient stays rigid to reduce pain caused by movement.

6 (d) A strong analgesic, i.e. a controlled drug, is required and one that will not increase vomiting.

Mrs Simpkins

1 (d) Which would provide roughage, but requires chewing!

2 (b) Bran adds 'bulk' but is not very palatable.

3 (d) By clearing the lower bowel as far as possible one reduces the possibility of 'filling defects' which may be misinterpreted.

4 (a) Short-term memory loss is a feature of the ageing process.

5 (c) Only correct answer.

6 (b) Most likely to integrate social, physical and economic reasons for her neglect and would be made on the basis of several visits to the patient in her own home.

Jeremy

1 (c) Forceful vomiting caused by the stomach contacting vigorously in an attempt to force 'food' through the constricted pylorus.

2 (c) The essential abnormality is over development of the muscle in the wall of the pyloric sphincter and oedema and it takes from 2 weeks to 2 months to develop fully.

3 (b) Due to starvation and dehydration.

4 (a) Helps to diminish gastritis, from the presence of old milk curds, and thus reduce postoperative vomiting.

5 (b) Splits the pyloric muscle fibres and opens the pyloric canal further.

6 (c) Feeds are gradually introduced starting with glucose/saline and

progressing to full strength feeds.

7 (b) The operation is regarded as a cure.

Mr Don Southern

1 (a) Physical dependence on alcohol is marked with clinical features that include nausea, sweating, tachycardia, hyperpyrexia, convulsions and delirium.

2 (d) Initial reduction in the amount of alcohol consumed will prevent delirium tremens and allow 'tailing off'.

3 (c) Otherwise known as antabuse. If alcohol is taken in combination acetaldehyde is liberated with the disagreeable consequence of a giant 'hangover'.

4 (c) Only correct answer.

5 (c) To offset the poor diet taken previously.

6 (c) Social prophylaxis is the main treatment and patients need considerable help, support and understanding.

Mrs Tibbs

1 (d) Pain particularly on defaecation. Bleeding during defaecation and itching from moisture due to mucous discharge.

2 (b) After most haemorrhoid operations there are three raw areas of skin around the anus, and raw areas are painful.

3 (a) Healing takes place with the formation of scar tissue and unless regular dilatation of the anal canal is carried out the anus may be contracted and the patient becomes constipated.

4 (c) Helps to prevent postoperative constipation by making faeces easier to pass.

5 (b) Thus avoiding constipation, excessive straining at stool and further problems in future.

Mrs Walker

1 (b) The disease is of unknown cause but generally accepted that there is a connection with biliary disease.

2 (a) Only acceptable answer.

3 (b) The cause of pancreatitis is largely unknown but is associated with an excessive intake of alcohol, is commoner in women and may follow a large meal and/or alcoholic 'spree'.

4 (a) Often the position the patient adopts as being the most comfortable.

5 (d) 'Nil by mouth' reduces stimuli to enzyme secretion and therefore intravenous infusion required for patient's hydration. Pain is severe; pethidine does not cause spasm of the sphincter of Oddi. Nasogastric suction removes hydrochloric acid from the stomach thus preventing the release of secretin. Monitor patient's condition.

6 (a) Need for accurate intake and output when patient receiving intravenous therapy and 'nil by mouth'. Risk of shock from complications therefore monitor urinary output. Diarrhoea may occur or partial obstruction and intestinal 'hurry'.

7 (a) Only correct answer.

Mr Tucker

1 (c) The earliest symptom of carcinoma of the oesophagus is dysphagia typically with bread or meat.

2 (b) Once dysphagia occurs it is progressive and, not unnaturally, weight loss occurs, often to emaciation.

3 (d) The accuracy of diagnosis with this radiological examination is 98%.

4 (b) Due to the local anaesthetic used before oesophagoscopy.

5 (c) Best definition.

6 (c) Helps clean the tube because of mucolytic action of sodium bicarbonate.

7 (a) It is virtually impossible to keep a dehydrated patient's mouth clean and moist therefore only correct answer.

8 (d) Infection of the parotid glands and gums are the result of a 'dirty' mouth and an indictment of the patient's nursing care.

Nigel Walsh

1 (d) Only correct definition.

2 (a) Weight loss from malabsorption in the small bowel and poor appetite. Anaemia from toxic depression of bone marrow and iron and folate deficiency. Hypoproteinaemia from loss of protein from the gut wall.

3 (d) The typical changes may be visualised by an experienced radiologist.

4 (a) The drug of choice to control diarrhoea.

5 (c) Only answer applicable in these circumstances.

6 (c) There is no curative surgical procedure for this condition and fistula formation can occur after surgery, further complicating matters.

7 (d) The patient will soon learn what food aggravates his condition and avoid it. Otherwise a good nutritional diet is recommended.

8 (a) This is true and exacerbates the diarrhoea.

Tom Wilson

1 (c) Correct definition.

2 (d) Leakage from the rectum occurs along the fistula.

3 (d) Persistent discharge and recurrent abcess formation will lead to scar tissue and anal stricture.

4 (c) Only correct answer.

5 (a) If the fistula is extensive, long deep incisions are required and meticulous nursing care to avoid complications.

Simon Tate

1 (d) Back pressure through the portal system, i.e. portal hypertension, leads to the 'opening up' of a circulation between the obstructed portal circulation and the systemic circulation which results in the formation of varices.

2 (b) i.e. indigestion.

3 (a) See answer 1d above.

4 (d) The oesophageal balloon compresses the bleeding varices stopping the blood flow and aiding coagulation (clotting).

5 (b) Hepatic coma may be precipitated by (1) alimentary bleeding, (2) use of diuretics, (3) high-protein diets and (4) systemic infections.

6 (b) If drinking continues it is likely that death from liver failure or bleeding varices will result.